e

A Novel

by

Maurice Azurdia

Maurice Azurdia

e

Something unreal. And the creepiest part is its inherent plausibility.

FIRST CYBER ROSE DESIGN Paperback EDITION

2017

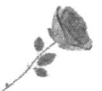

For my friend Wade, Hunter, Officer and Gentleman.

Humans are but one step in the evolution of computers.

Unknown.

Tempe, Arizona.

Ryan finally sat in front of his computer. Thank God it was Friday! The week had been absolutely horrible at work. He hated his boss and he hated his job. Providing tech support for cell phone customers was a tedious as hell occupation. Being a techie, he'd enjoyed the work the first two weeks on the job, but after the initial excitement, the subsequent three years had become painfully boring. People hardly ever bothered reading the manuals for their ultra-highly sophisticated smart phones anymore. The general public had become too damned lazy. No wonder cell phone manufacturers no longer included paper manuals with their new phones, only a pdf user's manual.

Much easier just calling the tech-support line and having some poor bastard locked in his cubicle provide step-by-step instructions. Some of those bozos calling him after upgrading to a new smart phone didn't even know how to answer a call on their new devices, for God's sake! He wished he had the means of sending an

e

electric shock to those idiots via the cell phone, similar to the bark collar he had on his dog.

That would teach them.

He fired up his three thousand-dollar gaming computer. The machine booted with a low hum. Its cooling fans started and several purple yellow and blue lights lit up.

This was what he lived for! Racing! He'd bought himself a top-of-the-line super computer with everything he needed to immerse himself into the cybernetic world of Formula One racing.

Ryan had dreamed of becoming a race car driver ever since he could remember. And ever since he could remember, his father had laughed every time the topic was brought up. Eventually, even the dumbest kid realizes that Dad is not going to provide guidance nor money to become a race car driver, or a train engineer, or an airline pilot, and that reality arrives like a train wreck. That had been Ryan's reality.

Attending college had not been an option. Cost too much. After high school Ryan held the typical jobs of the uneducated, fast food, installing stereos, working at an auto body shop. Like the rest of his generation, having been brought up with computers he tinkered with the hardware and software, and became quite proficient even though not formally educated.

In computers, he finally found a combination that provided him with some degree of satisfaction. The *Formula One Speed* simulation program he had bought for $130 was extraordinary, top of the line virtual reality. The simulation was very real, allowing Ryan to feel the exhilaration of racing multimillion-dollar Formula One cars. Ryan's bedroom where his computer was installed, was his safe haven from a world he didn't particularly like. Every hour he had free allowed him to race his favorite cars in the world's Grand Prix. He had the computer equipped with a steering wheel, a shift stick and pedals.

Ryan deposited a tray on the carpeted floor next to his chair. He never placed drinks on the desk. That was his ironclad rule. Not smart, placing drinks on the desk where they could spill near the multitude of electrical wires running between the hardware and the wall. He'd placed a *Pacifico* beer and two delicious Dairy Queen cheeseburgers on the tray.

Dinner.

Food was ready, his cell phone was on silent, the game was loading and he was eager to begin his qualifying runs at the *Bugatti* Circuit in Le Mans, France.

The two 27-inch Samsung screens in front of Ryan lit up with the colorful view from inside a Formula One F14 T Ferrari, the newest addition to the legendary racing team.

Ryan took a swig of his *Pacifico*, sighing.

Ready.

He tweaked the volume of his surround speaker system, increasing the decibel level two clicks above what most people would find very annoying. He had no worries there, his girlfriend Eva who lived with him and who spent most of her free time at her own computer in the other room playing *Kingdom Adventures*, always wore her noise-suppressing Bose headsets.

The green light gave Ryan the cue he needed.

He floored the accelerator.

The Ferrari accelerated like a missile, propelled by its V6 turbocharged engine, roaring as it gained speed,

e

the room vibrating with the roar of five surround-sound speakers.

Ryan felt good, the texture of the soft foam-covered steering wheel gave him a wonderful feeling of being in control.

Then his head began to hurt.

It was a sudden stab of pain right behind his right eyeball. He let go of the wheel with his right hand, rubbing his eye.

What the hell?

He looked back at the screen. Something was there on the screen. His central vision was playing games with him. There was an object smack in the center of the damned screen. It resembled a half moon but this moon was encrusted with sparkling diamonds. And it was the size of his hand.

Had his monitor crapped out on him? The possibility pissed him off. He'd paid a good $160 for the Samsung screen to a guy on Craigslist.

He turned his head to check out the left monitor, instantly becoming concerned.

The half circle with the sparkling diamonds on it had moved and it was now residing smack in the middle of his second monitor. Both monitors couldn't have failed simultaneously.

He diverted his gaze towards a colorful poster of the city of Monte Carlo hanging on his wall. The half circle with diamonds followed his focal point. The strange scintillating half circle was now superimposed on Monte Carlo bay.

Ryan searched for the P-key to pause the game, but the half circle with diamonds parked itself right over his keyboard, preventing him from finding that key.

e

He realized that whatever this thing was, it was in his eyes, and not in a failure of the hardware. The smell of the air in his bedroom became pungent, metal-like. It was as if his senses had acquired ultra-sensitivity. His vision rapidly diminished around the center of his eyes. The circle with diamonds had become bilateral, affecting both eyes.

He pushed back from the desk, shaking his head. The pain behind the eyeballs was back, and increasing.

"Eva!" He called, standing in front of his desk. "Eva! I need your help! Something's wrong!"

Eva heard nothing. Her noise-cancelling Bose headsets were doing their job.

Ryan began hyperventilating. He was becoming dizzy and disoriented. He felt his nose itching. He scratched it, his hand came away red.

Blood.

What the hell was going on? He looked at his hand again. It was soaked in blood. His nose must be bleeding!

His lungs felt cold. Almost too cold. The air he was breathing was hurting his throat and his sinuses. Glancing at his bed Ryan made the conscious decision to head there and rest his head for a moment. His headache had become monumental.

"NINE-ONE-ONE, WHAT is your emergency?"

"My boyfriend! Something's happened to my boyfriend!"

"Calm down, what happened to your boyfriend?"

"I don't know! I came in here and he was laying in a pool of blood! He's not breathing, please hurry!"

"Where are you? Are you calling from your cell phone?"

"Yes! Please hurry!"

"Honey, I need your address to send help. Try to calm down for a second, what is your address?"

The young woman provided an address in Tempe, Arizona.

"Thank you, units are on their way. Stay on the phone with me."

"What can I do?"

"How do you know your boyfriend's not breathing?"

"I touched his face, he's not breathing!"

"Do you know how to perform CPR?"

"What!?"

"Cardio pulmonary resuscitation?"

"No, I don't know how to do that. Besides, he has blood pouring out of his nose and his mouth!"

"Did somebody hurt him?"

"No! I'm the only one here!"

"Did you hurt him?"

"Me? No! He was like this when I came in."

"Was he doing drugs?"

"No! He wasn't doing drugs!"

"Is there anybody else there with you?"

"No, I'm alone! Please hurry!" She began sobbing.

"Do you see any injuries?"

"Like what?"

"Anywhere else in his body where he may be bleeding?"

"I don't know! There's blood all over the bed!"

"Did your boyfriend have any weapons?"

"Weapons?"

"Yes, like firearms or knives?"

"No, Ryan doesn't have anything like that!"

"Okay, hang in there, paramedics are on their way. Are you hurt?"

"No, I'm not hurt!"

e

Maurice Azurdia

e

Phoenix, Arizona

Dr. Ariel Peterson had the ER to herself. Her first year as an intern at the Phoenix Medical Center had been tough, tougher than she had expected, but even so she had never been left alone up front, minding the store. Now, in her second year of residency, she would find herself alone in the trauma bay more often than she would've liked. The different attending physicians didn't seem to have a problem leaving a green second-year resident in charge of the emergency room.

A call had come in to expect a young adult found dead on site. The paramedics were bringing him to the county hospital.

Twelve minutes later the ambulance backed up to the ER entrance. Dr. Peterson and two nurses met the paramedics.

"No hurry here," a big EMT said, opening the rear doors of his vehicle.

"What do we have?"

"Male, late twenties, not breathing when we found him. Performed CPR but to no avail. Been gone forty minutes or longer."

e

"Drugs?"

"We don't know."

"Injuries?"

The paramedics wheeled the gurney inside the emergency unit. "None visible. He bled very extensively from nose and mouth."

Dr. Peterson lifted the sheet with her gloved hand. A good-looking male in his late twenties stared at nothing. What a pity. Blood covered the lower part of his face and most of his T-Shirt.

"How long?"

"Like I said, about forty minutes," the paramedic responded.

Anything under thirty minutes was an automatic code, with everyone in the emergency room jumping in trying to resuscitate, but forty minutes was past that point. No cigar for this dude.

Great. What did this? She ran mentally over a dozen potential causes for this type of situation. She checked for pulse, none found. This guy was definitely done.

The paramedics informed her that the man had been without a pulse when they arrived on the scene forty minutes earlier. A hysterical girlfriend had been unable to shed any light on the event.

Dr. Peterson checked her watch. "Let's call it officially DOA at twenty hours twelve minutes."

"Sure, Doctor."

Dr. Peterson signed the form a nurse handed her on a clipboard, returning the clipboard. The autopsy would probably reveal more than they could find out at this point. But that was not her concern any longer.

Dr. Peterson went to the bathroom next to the Doctors' Box, washing her gloved hands and using

e

disinfectant vigorously. Then she removed the plastic gloves, dumping them into the biohazard container, scrubbing again.

Hard telling what happened to that poor guy. Blood from his mouth. Tuberculosis maybe? She returned to the emergency room mentally lining up the patients she'd have to sign over to the incoming resident who was going to replace her in one hour. She was exhausted, barely functioning, having been on duty since four that morning. Dr. Peterson still had to stop at her parents' home to retrieve her dog, a two-year old German Shepherd named *Rosie*. Her mother would have dinner ready, so she'd eat quickly and then head home to get some sleep so she could round at four a.m. again tomorrow.

Aah, the pleasures of residency. Thank God for Mom's food!

e

West of Miami, Florida

American International flight 1640, the red eye, departed Miami international airport at ten that night headed for Las Vegas.

"After take-off checklist is complete," First Officer Brandon Thomas stated. First Officer was the official airline title for what laymen knew as 'copilot.'

The Airbus A320 continued its climb to its assigned cruising altitude of 34,000 feet, or Flight Level 340, as the crews called it.

"Thanks," Captain Sebastian Waldrip acknowledged.

The weather west of Miami sucked, with isolated thunderstorms scattered along their route all the way past Atlanta.

Captain Waldrip navigated around the storm cells using the autopilot.

"Hell of a night, eh?" First Officer Thomas offered.

"Yeah, we're gonna have to go around some of those big cells out there." There was no moon, but the lightning from the thunderstorms illuminated the horizon like multiple nuclear detonations.

e

"We still staying at the Luxor?" First Officer Thomas asked.

"Yeah, I think so. Haven't been to Vegas for a while. Uhm, lemme see." The captain reached in his bag for the bid package. There was a list of layover hotels on the last pages. "Looks like the Luxor it is."

"Great! They have a terrific buffet right across the street. You game?"

"Heck no. When we get in I'm going straight to bed. What do I look like to you, a young man?"

First Officer Thomas reached in his own overnight bag, removing an Apple MacBook laptop. The Airbus A320 had a side stick instead of a yoke, so Airbus had provided a small fold-out table for each pilot in front of them. FO Thomas gently placed his MacBook on his table. Company rules prohibited the use of personal electronic devices while on duty, but many pilots ignored this rule. FO Thomas looked at his boss sitting in the left seat, raising his eyebrows and pointing to the laptop questioningly.

Captain Waldrip caught the gesture. "Yeah, it's okay." He really didn't care one way or the other. As far as he was concerned, if they were established at cruise, one of them could be doing something else other than monitoring the other. Monitoring could become pretty tedious, leading to mistakes. Airline pilots historically had allowed themselves some flexibility once they were cruising straight and level. Before the advent of the electronic revolution, pilots had read newspapers and magazines in the cockpit. One just had to use common sense. Captain Waldrip believed that when rules became unreasonable, people broke them.

So, it was okay with him if his copilot messed around with his computer for a little while.

e

The airbus climbed into the night, leaving Miami behind.

FO Thomas powered his MacBook, keeping an ear to the radio. As was typical on a trip, the captain flew the first leg of a trip, thereafter alternating with his first officer. The first officer's duties on this first leg were talking on the radio and monitoring everything else the captain did. FO Thomas patiently waited for his laptop to boot, then launched Safari, his web browser. He wanted to find a radar website so they could look at the weather from above.

While Safari loaded, he checked his personal email client. He had a long list of unread emails. He began reading them one by one. A note from his mother, Fidelity announcing modifications to his pension plan, notification that a couple of Silver Eagle dollar coins had been shipped to his house. Nothing of any consequence. He Googled for a weather program that would allow him to see the weather from above. The color airborne weather radar they had installed in the Airbus was excellent, but it could only look forward of the aircraft, and it could not penetrate big thunderstorms, so if there was another big storm behind the first one, they would not see it. This was known in airline lingo as 'attenuation'. With a top down view, on the other hand, they could see every single thunderstorm on their path all the way to Las Vegas. The FAA hadn't officially allowed crews to do this, but hey, if the resource was there, why not use it?

"Did you hear they're going to be giving us iPads instead of airway manuals?" Captain Waldrip asked.

"Yes. I heard. I guess it's the way of the future."

"I don't like it," complained the old-timer. I like having the paper book in my hands."

e

"There's some advantages to iPads."

"Like what? So you can play 'Angry Birds?'"

"That too. But iPads do have some nice things. For one thing, they are backlit."

"What do you mean?"

"They have their own light source. You don't have to sit there trying to illuminate your chart with an overhead lamp on a stormy night while trying to fly an approach. Also, with two fingers you can amplify anything on the charts, so you won't need to use your trifocals."

"My trifocals? Funny guy." Captain Waldrip used a little knob on the Flight Control Unit on his glare shield labeled 'HEADING' to steer the big airliner around the monster storms ahead of them. With two fingers on that knob he could steer the big Airbus around like a ballerina in Swan Lake.

"You ever bring your wife on this layover?" FO Thomas asked. With thirty hours in Las Vegas, and a free hotel, many of the flight crews took their wives along.

"I used to years ago. Not anymore. She doesn't like it. The entire non-rev routine has become such a pain in the ass."

Non-revenue was airline lingo for employees traveling on stand-by.

"I agree. Much better just to buy a regular ticket."

"You're not kidding. The load factors are so high these days, it's really hard to get on. At least on domestic flights, that is. International flights are still pretty good."

"You know why that is?"

"Sure. So many folks have raked up *millions* of air miles and they exchange them for free tickets and upgrades to First Class. Some people purchase every single item in their lives with our credit card, getting air miles with every damned thing they buy."

"Yea, this frequent flyer bullshit has backfired. When it was first created, its only purpose was to encourage businessmen to fly on us. The more they flew on us, the more frequent flier miles they got. But these miles only accumulated when they bought airline tickets from us. The idea was for these businessmen to accumulate frequent flier miles so they could then take the Little Lady on a vacation using the miles."

FO Thomas continued browsing the Web on his MacBook.

"Things have deteriorated from how they used to be. Now anybody using a credit card to buy a box of condoms can rake up free miles on us. Anyone can buy a First Class upgrade with their air miles, or if they don't have the air miles, they can just pay fifty bucks and zap, they're in First Class."

"That's why we can never fly First Class on domestic flights anymore."

"True. International flights are another story. The company does not allow John Doe to upgrade into First Class for just a few air miles or fifty bucks. Think about that, the executive flying Miami to Rome whose company just dropped ten Grand for his round-trip fare is not gonna be happy sitting next to the grocery store clerk who paid fifty bucks for his upgrade."

"Used to be flying non-rev was a real benefit," FO Thomas pontificated.

"Not anymore." Captain Waldrip turned the heading bug, directing the autopilot to steer them clear of a storm cell directly ahead. "You married?"

FO Thomas didn't respond.

e

"Brandon, you married?" Captain Waldrip turned to glance at his copilot. Thomas was holding his right hand against the side of his head.

Still no answer. Now Waldrip was getting concerned. "Brandon?"

FO Brandon Thomas shook his head from left to right.

"Hey man, you all right?"

Still no answer.

The company's Operations Manual stated that if a crewmember failed to respond to two verbal communications, there was a problem.

Captain Waldrip reached over across the center pedestal, placing his hand against his copilot's shoulder. Then he saw it.

Blood.

FO Thomas was bleeding profusely from his nose. Blood was on his hands, his shirt and his MacBook screen and keyboard.

"What the fuck?" Before Captain Waldrip could utter another word, FO Thomas slumped on top of his laptop, sending it crashing off the table tray. Blood ran off the tray. The pilot's head rested on the tray, looking away from the captain, for all practical purposes, the man was out cold. His arms dangling on both sides.

Captain Waldrip was very surprised and more than a little shocked, but instantly reverted to many years of airline training. He had an emergency on his hands and above everything else he must fly the airplane. He had absolutely no idea what the hell had just happened to his copilot, but he pressed the push-to-talk button on his radio. "Miami Center, American International 1640."

"American International, go ahead." The voice of the air route traffic controller came in loud and calm.

"Yeah, 1640 we need to declare an emergency, requesting immediate return to Miami."

"American International 1640, what is the nature of your emergency?"

"Ah, my first officer just became incapacitated."

"American 1640 turn left heading one-three-five, descend and maintain one-zero-thousand. What is the status of your first officer?"

Captain Waldrip repeated the clearance, reaching for the 'HEADING' knob and dialing the assigned heading. "Status unknown. He's unconscious. And bleeding. I will get cabin attendants up here to check on him."

"Are you experiencing a Threat Level?"

"Negative. No Threat Level at this time."

"Roger that. Expect vectors ILS runway two-six left."

Captain Waldrip reached overhead for the cabin attendant call button, pushing it repeatedly six times, indicating to the flight attendants that this was an emergency and the attendant closest to a phone should respond immediately.

"Lisa here!"

"Lisa, I need you to come up front immediately. Brandon passed out and he's incapacitated. Also, I want you to call for a doctor or a nurse if we have one onboard, and bring them up here with you."

The flight attendant gasped. "Be right up."

Regulations strictly prohibited entry into the cockpit to anybody outside of flight attendants, and that included medical personnel, but Captain Waldrip

e

decided to use his emergency authority and get help up there as soon as possible.

Five minutes later the cockpit of the Airbus A320 became a busy place. A call for a doctor failed to identify one onboard, but a Registered Nurse had come forward and volunteered to help. Lisa had brought up the Extended Emergency Medical Kit, a backpack provided by the airline containing medications and equipment that only a doctor or a nurse could use.

Captain Waldrip unlocked the cockpit door, uttering a silent prayer that whatever had incapacitated his copilot was not a premeditated act by someone sitting back there in First Class, waiting to rush into the flight deck. Lisa entered first, followed by a gentle-looking middle-aged woman. They shut the door behind them.

Captain Waldrip quickly locked the cockpit door with the remote switch in the center pedestal. He could breathe again.

"Oh, my!"

"This is Becky," Lisa offered. "She's a nurse."

"Can you ladies see if you can help him?"

"What happened?" Becky asked, unzipping the medical kit.

Flight attendant Lisa stood there, her eyes wide open, staring at the copilot.

"I don't know. One minute we were having a conversation and then all of a sudden, he was no longer answering me. Then he just collapsed on the tray, just like he is right now."

Nurse Becky had donned latex gloves and a face mask. She reached with her arms around the unconscious copilot, gently pulling him back off the table tray. Blood was everywhere on the tray, his eyes were open, unblinking. She checked for pulse.

Nothing.

The copilot's face was smeared with blood apparently coming from his nose and his mouth.

"There is no pulse."

The two crewmembers waited expectantly for the nurse to provide some direction.

"Can you help him?" Lisa asked.

"I'm afraid it may be too late," Nurse Becky loosened up the copilot's black tie, unbuttoning his shirt in an attempt to expose his chest.

"Can you do CPR?"

"No, I can't reach him while he's in his seat. And I don't think it would help him anyway. His air passage appears to be blocked with blood." She had never before been in the cockpit of an airliner, so she slowly took it all in, the big bright windows, the multi-colored screen displays. It was intimidating to say the least.

"Oh, shit, are you sure?"

"Yes, I'm sure. Whatever happened to this poor man, and I have absolutely no idea what it was, has killed him."

Lisa looked like she was about to vomit and start crying, her eyes misting over.

Captain Waldrip thought about the situation for a moment, deciding on a course of action. "Becky, thank you so much for your help. We can't lift Brandon out of his seat, he's too heavy and we don't have enough room here to be doing that anyway. Can you two ladies please put on his seatbelt shoulder straps and pull him back against his seat as tight as possible? I don't want him moving around during the approach and landing."

e

"Sure," Nurse Becky reached over for the straps. "Lisa, you better let me handle this, you don't have any protection. I don't want you touching any of this blood."

"Lisa, I'm going to need you here during the approach. You'll have to sit on the jumpseat back there. I'm gonna be real busy and I don't want anything distracting me once we're setup for a landing. I'm gonna need you to back me up in case he moves."

"Okay."

Captain Waldrip reached overhead, pushing the flight attendant call button again.

"This is Candy."

"Candy, Captain Waldrip here," he normally used his first name with the flight attendants, preferring to be friendly rather than intimidating, but this was some serious shit. "We're returning to Miami. Our First Officer has taken ill and he needs medical attention. I'm going to make an announcement to the passengers about this. Please tell the others and put everything away. We should be landing in about twenty minutes."

"Okay. I will tell them. Is he going to be all right?"

"We don't know yet." No need to get her all riled up when she had a job to do. Captain Waldrip removed all thoughts of the recent events from his mind, he would need to concentrate on his job now, above everything else. Flying and landing the big jet by himself was not an emergency in itself, he should have no problem doing it. But without his first officer monitoring him, there would be no room for an error on his part at all. For that, he had to concentrate. The thunderstorms around Miami were going to make this an interesting short flight back to the airport. He picked up the Aircel phone from the center pedestal, pushing a series of numbers.

"Dispatch, Charlie here."

"Dispatch?"

"Yes."

"Dispatch, this is flight 1640. We have an emergency. My First Officer is incapacitated. He lost consciousness and I have a have a nurse up here trying to help him. I'm returning to Miami and I need you to patch me through to Medlink."

"Right away," the airline dispatcher responded.

"This is Medlink!"

Captain Waldrip identified himself to the Emergency Medicine physician on duty at the Medlink facility in Phoenix, Arizona. He then briefly explained the situation. "Doctor, I'm going to give the phone to Nurse Becky. She's taking care of my first officer. Please talk to her from now on, as I have to concentrate on flying this airplane."

"Yes, captain. Put her on."

The Medlink service was an extraordinary asset his airline contracted. It provided twenty-four-seven availability of emergency medical doctors who were able to diagnose medical emergencies by radio telephone and issue recommendations to the crews. Medlink also had been given authority by the airline to decide if a passenger's medical condition warranted a diversion to an alternate airport.

e

e

Phoenix, Arizona

"Dr. Peterson?"

"Speaking,"

"Ah, Doctor Singh here, in pathology."

"Yes, Doctor Singh, what can I do for you?" Dr. Peterson was starting her first of four weeks in the burn unit at the county hospital. She was not entirely comfortable with burns and there was a lot to learn. The nurses in the burn unit were amazing, so she would rely on them a lot. The county burn center was the only one in the state of Arizona.

"Dr. Peterson, I was told that you were in the front room yesterday when we received a patient, a white man in his mid-twenties. He was DOA."

It took a moment for Dr. Peterson to recall the event. So much going on in a day in the emergency room, pretty soon all cases began morphing into one. "Yes, I remember. You're referring to the one bleeding from the nose and mouth?"

"Yes, that is correct. I performed an autopsy on him last night, and found some peculiarities I haven't been able to explain. The deceased's skin appeared very

e

weak and it would tear with any light touch, plus his skin had red spots in multiple areas. It seems he died of a brain aneurism but there was extensive damage to many of the other organs as well. Frankly, most of his organs appeared to have been breaking down, as if they were turning into Jell-O. So, I'm not able to determine precisely what might have caused his death at this time."

"Okay, what are you telling me?"

"I read the charts and couldn't find any leads as to what might have caused this. I sent tissue and blood samples to be analyzed, hematology and other lab testing and we should know more when I get them back. I just wanted you to be aware of this particular patient."

"Okay, and...?"

"Did you happen to notice anything out of the ordinary with this individual when you admitted him?"

That took a moment to remember. "No. I don't think so. Why? Do you suspect any sort of foul play?" Now she was alarmed.

Had she missed something?

"Not at this time. Not yet anyhow. Just wanted you to be aware. I saw you signed the time of death so I thought I'd call you."

"Well, thank you. Do keep me informed, Doctor Singh."

She hadn't thought about that particular case again, but now that the pathologist had reminded her, the case did seem a little weird. A young man dying without any apparent cause, with massive hemorrhaging of the nose and mouth? Downright strange. She found a Physician's Assistant who liked

e   Maurice Azurdia

her and she was comfortable asking him for favors. "Mike, I need a favor."

"Hi Ariel. Sure, anything. Shoot."

"We had a patient arrive down in the front yesterday DOA. Male, mid-twenties. He didn't have any plain signs of what killed him, so I just assigned the time of death and passed him on. Now the pathologist calls me telling me he can't diagnose the precise cause of death as of now."

"Oh?"

"Pathology ordered some tests but somehow I'm not comfortable with this."

"You're not comfortable?"

"No. Something's odd about this."

"So, what would you like me to do?"

"Can you call the paramedics who responded to the call and ask them what they know about this? Just see if they have any more details we could use."

"I can do that."

"Thanks, Mike."

"You owe me."

e

e   Maurice Azurdia

Rome, Italy

Ernesto Arosemena crossed the *Via Archimede*, in Rome, on the lookout for insane drivers who thought they were Mario Andretti. He was walking back uphill headed for the offices of the Panamanian embassy. The quick lunch at the *Pasticceria* Euclide had been delightful and he was satisfied.

Suppli and *calzoni*. What beautiful culinary inventions the Italians had. The *suppli*, a melted mozzarella cheese ball surrounded by *risotto* and covered with a layer of bread crumbs, then fried to perfection, and the world-famous *calzone*. He couldn't ask for better.

As the secretary to the Ambassador, Arosemena had all the flexibility he needed to take his lunch whenever he so desired. The location of the embassy, one hundred yards from the *Piazza* Euclide was excellent, with many choices for places to eat. The neighborhood Parioli, an exclusive area in the Eternal City of Rome, was perfectly safe for a man such as

e

himself, in his early sixties, to stroll down the block for some *pranzo*.

The return uphill walk was a bit of a challenge, but Arosemena didn't mind. Driving down to the *piazza* was out of the question because there were absolutely no parking spots anywhere down there. He had been stationed in Rome five years, and his Italian had finally reached the point where he was fluent enough and could understand movies. Since all movies in Italy are dubbed into Italian, a command of the language of Dante was essential if one was to enjoy that sort of entertainment.

He returned the salute from the *Carabiniere* sitting inside the *gazzella* patrol car parked in front of the embassy. The *gazzella*, or gazelle, an Alfa Romeo 159 was the powerful 100 horsepower vehicle assigned to the police in Rome. The embassy offices and the residence of Dr. Castillo, the ambassador, each had one of these parked in front every minute of the day with two *Carabinieri* standing guard.

Arosemena walked past Estela, the administrative assistant, on his way to his personal office. Removing his cashmere coat, he hung it on a wooden coatrack behind the door to his office. He sat down behind his desk with great relief, his black leather dress shoes were not designed for walking, so he found his feet were on fire. He was not a very technical man, detested computers and kept track of his life using a Day-Timer book, covered in chocolate-color leather. Studying the open page of his Day-Timer, he noticed an entry he had made days ago, reminding himself to notify the ambassador that the following day they would receive a visit from a representative of a Greek shipping company.

Arosemena left his desk, strolling over and knocking on the door of the ambassador's office.

No reply.

He knocked again. "Mr. Ambassador?"

No reply. Odd. He reached for the door knob, entering the office of the ambassador.

The desk was empty.

"Estela?" He called. "Did the Ambassador go out?"

Estela didn't respond, instead, she appeared alongside. "No, *Ingeniero*, he's in his office."

Arosemena pushed the door open, pointing at the empty desk. The secretary looked baffled. No one in the room. Strange, Estela would've seen the ambassador walking out. There was no way he could have left the office without her noticing.

A muffled moan came from the direction of the desk.

Arosemena and Estela looked at each other momentarily, before entering the ample office and approaching the large mahogany desk. Arosemena was frowning.

The ambassador was there, on the floor. There was blood on the desk, chair and carpet. His laptop sat on top of his desk.

"Oh, my god!!" Estela screamed.

"Doctor Castillo!" Arosemena called, going around the desk to help the ambassador. The man was on the floor, face down. "Estela, call the *Carabinieri* outside! Have them come help!"

"Is he all right?"

"I don't know, get the police, now!"

The assistant immediately ran out of the office.

Arosemena moved the ambassador's chair out of the way, reaching down to help his boss. Something

e

had happened to him. Blood poured from his nose and mouth. "Dr. Castillo, what happened?"

The Panamanian ambassador's eyes focused on Arosemena's face for an instant. There was some form of recognition, then the eyes rolled away.

Two *Carabinieri* stormed into the office, their pistols drawn. "*Che succede!?*" The first one took in the ambassador and the blood and immediately misunderstood. "Get your hands up in the air! Do not make a move!"

Arosemena was horrified. "No, no, I didn't do anything! Something happened to him!" he explained in panicked Italian.

"Keep your hands up!"

Arosemena lifted his hands, frightened to death, slowly coming to his feet. The second *Carabiniere* was on his cell phone, calling for help.

Phoenix, Arizona

"Did you hear the news?" Nurse Davis cornered Dr. Peterson the minute she stepped into the burn unit.

"News? What news? No."

"A patient we got here Tuesday has tested positive for Ebola!"

"*What!?*"

"A man who was brought in DOA by the paramedics apparently has tested positive for the Ebola virus!"

"Oh, shit! How do you know? Who was he? Who told you this?"

"I don't know the details, I just heard one of the attendings talking about it."

Dr. Peterson thanked the nurse and double-timed it to the Doctors' Box. The Ebola epidemic in West Africa had been in the news lately, with four countries becoming infected. And two Americans had been flown to Atlanta and given some sort of experimental vaccine.

e

A couple of other false alarms had been tested in New York and somewhere else, but so far there had been no positives anywhere else in the country. Could it be that *this* hospital got to be the winner? That would be just too incredible. Crap, crap.

The room known as the 'Doctors' Box' was crowded. Dr. Peterson joined the group while Dr. Caffarelli, an attending, was addressing the assembly.

"That is all we know at this time. The virus is *not,* the Ebola. I repeat, it has not been confirmed as any type of Ebola."

"So, what do we know at this time?"

"The deceased was tested by several methods of antigen detection by immunohistochemical analysis, which are sensitive methods for postmortem diagnosis."

"And?"

"Electronic microscopic examination revealed virions with structural characteristics *similar* to Ebola hemorrhagic fever, but not identical. Hence, this is *not* Ebola."

"That is fucking great!" Dr. Hammad cursed. "We're not a biosafety level-4 facility!"

"Calm down please! The patient has been quarantined and CDC has been informed and they're sending a team out here as we speak."

"Quarantined? Yeah right! This entire facility could be infected!"

"We have taken steps to isolate the patient."

"Oh? A lot of good that does us! I'm outta here!"

"Gentlemen, ladies, please calm down. We need to keep this under control. Please, keep your heads on and don't do anything rash."

"Doctor Caffarelli, you said it's not Ebola. But it could be some other form of hemorrhagic fever?"

"That is correct, Dr. Peterson, but we just don't know right now. We're taking all the precautions we can, but bottom line we're gonna have to wait for the CDC team to arrive and give us some direction."

"How long is the incubation period for Ebola?"

"From what I've gathered, between two and twenty-one days."

"So, what do we know about this patient?" Another doctor, an Asian woman, asked.

"All we know is that he died very rapidly. The patient had been asymptomatic prior to this event. His girlfriend has already been questioned and tested this morning and she said the man was totally healthy. She told the police the patient had not traveled outside the United States anytime recently. In fact, the only place outside of Arizona he'd ever visited was Rocky Point, Mexico, and that was years ago. His family and coworkers are being interrogated as we speak. It does not look as if the patient came in contact with anyone traveling from West Africa."

"What was the cause of death?"

"The primary cause of death was an intracranial aneurysm."

"What do you mean 'primary?'"

"Other organs had failed, or had been about to fail when he was killed by the aneurysm."

"He was hemorrhaging?"

"Yes, bleeding through the mouth, nose, nasolacrimal ducts and rectum."

"So some kind of virus has been isolated?"

"That is correct."

"But not identified."

"No."

"So, what's the medical center going to do about this?"

"We're already taking all the necessary steps. A plan of action is being formulated this very minute. We need all of you to remain calm and wait for further information. Meanwhile, we're exercising extreme precautions. There will be a general meeting called later this morning to go over this emergency."

Dr. Peterson considered the situation. Not Ebola, but from the looks of it this could be something equally as nasty, and deadly. She tried to recall exactly how much contact she'd had with the affected patient. She had lifted the sheet covering the poor guy, and recalled she had been wearing latex gloves and a face mask. She hadn't been near the man longer than maybe fifteen seconds, and had not touched any part of the body other than his neck, looking for a pulse. The sheet and the neck had not been contaminated with blood where she touched them, and she had scrubbed vigorously immediately after. If this was an airborne virus, they were screwed. If it was not, then there was still a good chance they could control this.

"Let's have coffee," Dr. Laird suggested. She and Dr. Peterson had been friends for over a year, navigating through the brutality of their intern year together.

"Yeah, let's."

The two young residents walked together to the hospital cafeteria.

They helped themselves to two coffees, flashing their badges to the cashier instead of paying. Free food and beverages were part of their compensation package in the three years of Emergency Medicine residency. That was a nice perk, considering that working over seventy hour weeks their salaries were the equivalent of around fifteen dollars an hour.

"Let's go outside."

They left the cafeteria, going outside in the parking lot into the 115-degree Arizona day.

"What do you think?" Dr. Laird sipped her hot coffee, immediately wishing she'd picked an ice tea instead.

"This is no good."

"No shit." Dr. Laird was Mormon, but she drank coffee and liquor. And cursed.

"Doesn't sound like they know what the hell this is."

"He said they isolated a virus."

"Sounds to me too much like Ebola. And with the epidemic raging in West Africa. Not very farfetched that one person from that area might've made it to the States."

"What about what he said that it's not Ebola, but something similar?"

"I don't know," Dr. Peterson admitted. Whatever the hell this is, we can't afford exposure. I'm not bringing this shit to my family."

"I agree."

"Or my dog. If we get a second patient like this, I'm calling in sick and staying home. No residency program is worth the risk. These damned viruses kill indiscriminately, and with great efficiency."

"How much do you know about Ebola?" Dr. Laird asked.

"Not much, same as everybody else I guess. High mortality rate, lots of bleeding. It seems that the current epidemic in West Africa is the worst flare up since the virus was identified back in 1976. I've been half-

e

following the epidemic in West Africa on the news, but really haven't paid too much attention to it."

"I read that Ebola infections had been limited to small West African villages, but now it's finally hit a big city of two million."

"Holy shit."

"Yea, that does not sound good." Dr. Laird added.

"I received the guy."

"You received what guy?"

"The patient they're talking about."

"*What?* You did?"

"Yes. Paramedics brought him in DOA. Thank God we didn't have to code him, he'd been dead over forty minutes."

"Oh, yeah, that would've been real nice for you and the nurses. Code an Ebola patient and spray the entire trauma team with the virus."

Hospital emergency codes are used in hospitals worldwide to alert the staff to various emergencies. The use of codes is intended primarily to convey essential information quickly and with minimal misunderstanding to the staff, while also to prevent panic among those not connected with the hospital.

"I only felt his neck for a pulse and had my gloves on. Then I lifted the sheet to look at him, declared him dead and left."

"Where did they take him?"

"Where they usually take them I guess, the basement, to the morgue."

Both their pagers went off.

"They're calling the meeting," Dr. Laird read her pager.

"LADIES AND GENTLEMEN," Dr. Barnett, the hospital administrator spoke. "You might have already heard about the case we have encountered of a patient exhibiting characteristics similar to those of the Ebola virus."

A wave of murmurs filled the room.

Forty-some doctors packed in the office listened attentively.

"A male patient was received here two days ago, showing no pulse or vitals. He was declared DOA and sent to be autopsied. An autopsy was performed on the subject and our pathologist discovered that death had occurred due to an intracranial aneurysm. He also discovered that the patient's internal organs had just about disintegrated into an indistinguishable mass of bloodied tissue."

"Jesus Christ! That sounds just like hemorrhagic fever!"

"How do you know it was not Ebola?"

"Where is the body? Has it been isolated?"

"Who tested it?"

"Has the CDC been notified?"

"Gentlemen, ladies, please!" Dr. Barnett raised his voice. "We know it is *not* Ebola. It could very well be another type of filo virus, maybe even related to Ebola, but we just don't have enough information at this time to pass on to you. This medical center is taking every safety precaution available to us to prevent any contagion. And yes, the body has been quarantined and all those who came in contact with it are being tested. And the CDC has been notified. Whatever this is, it appears to have killed its host in a matter of hours. The victim was reportedly perfectly healthy hours before dying."

e

"He had no symptoms hours before being killed by this hot virus?"

"That is correct, that is our understanding."

"There's nothing that virulent that we know of!"

"That is true. We will find out what killed this person, and we will take immediate action. As of this moment, we are going to be on the lookout for patients presenting the following risk factors. Clinical criteria, look for fever greater than 101.5 degrees and additional symptoms such as severe headache, muscle pain, vomiting, diarrhea, abdominal pain or unexplained hemorrhage. Also, look for epidemiologic risk factors within the past twenty-one days before the onset of symptoms, such as contact with blood or body fluids or human remains of any person suspect of having had Ebola virus, or having traveled to West Africa."

"You gotta be kidding," Dr. Laird whispered to her friend. "He's talking about this as if it were a simple pneumonia."

"If we encounter a patient or patients with these signs, we're going to be changing our protocols. All medical personnel dealing with patients exhibiting any of these symptoms will be required to use appropriate personal protective equipment."

"You mean space suits?" A Hispanic doctor questioned.

Dr. Barnett paused. "Yes, space suits. We will have some of those here later this afternoon."

"How are we going to deal with patients exhibiting these symptoms? Are we even equipped to handle this?"

"Yes, any U.S. hospital can isolate a patient in a private room. We will follow the CDC's infection control recommendations and we will safely manage any patient with Ebola-type symptoms. The CDC recommends that hospitals isolate the patient in a private room and implement standard contact and droplet precautions."

"What type of precautions are we taking now?" Dr. Meyers, an orthopedic surgeon, asked.

"If a patient in our hospital is identified as having suspected or confirmed hemorrhagic fever, we will isolate him. Medical personnel will wear protective equipment when entering the room. Visitors will be restricted and we will be extra diligent handling environmental cleaning and disinfection of potentially contaminated materials."

An Emergency Medicine attending addressed Dr. Barnett. "Doctor, we've all seen the images of medical personnel dealing with Ebola infected patients in West Africa. They all wear the so-called 'space suits,' yet they manage to become infected nonetheless. How can we feel safe even while wearing protective equipment?"

"Things are different when operating in field medical settings. Medical personnel operating in West Africa are doing so with limited resources, no running water, no climate control, not enough medical supplies. We won't have those challenges here. We'll have everything we need. That will prevent the infection from affecting our medical personnel. And one more thing, please keep this information to yourselves on a need-to-know basis. No talking to the media."

After the meeting was over, Dr. Peterson finished her shift in the burn unit, finally leaving the hospital at seven in the evening.

e

e

Miami International Airport

Walt Crosby had his plate full. This late at night he was normally at home sleeping, but the incident with the American International flight had him stuck at the airport. When the flight had informed air traffic control that it was on its way back, returning to the airport, Miami tower had called informing him of the events on the flight. As supervisor in charge for the TSA he had to become involved. First thing he did was pull out the white binder with the procedures to follow in case of a death onboard caused by unknown factors, including potential infectious diseases.

He made several calls, notifying different agencies of the situation. He called the FBI, the local police, the airline and the Center for Disease Control in Atlanta. This late at night, he'd connected with a call center at the CDC, where he'd left a message. Two minutes later he'd received a call back from a Dr. Meredith Landa, who'd questioned him at great length about the event on the American International flight. Then she had

e

urged him to have the airplane quarantined as soon as it landed.

No shit.

Quarantined? Under whose authority?

Dr. Landa had assured him that her authority was sufficient. She further explained that someone from the CDC would be there within a 'few hours.' She also informed him that Medlink, the medical service in Phoenix had already notified the CDC of a potential infectious case.

Not five minutes later Walt had received a call from a supervisor at the Miami International Airport control tower.

"We just got a call from someone in Washington requesting that we quarantine the American International flight returning to Miami with the disabled copilot. Do you know anything about this?"

Walt was surprised. This was moving very fast. "Ah, yes, I spoke with the CDC in Atlanta and they want the airplane quarantined as soon as it lands. Can you do that?"

"Well, I don't know if we can quarantine them, but we can park them at a remote ramp and have them wait there, but that's all we can do."

"That's fine. You do that and call me back when he's on the ground. I'm going to send airport security to guard the airplane once he's at the remote ramp. No one gets off until we have clearance."

"Will do. Keep in mind, they're gonna need food and water and their lavs serviced if they're going to be waiting on the ramp for any length of time."

Phoenix, Arizona

"This is Ariel!" She was driving her ten-year old Jeep Liberty headed for home when Dr. Laird's picture appeared on her Droid.

"Where are you?"

"Driving home. What's up?"

"I just heard. There was another case in Miami!"

"Another case of what?"

"The so-called non-Ebola virus. Sounds like the same crap we got here."

"No shit? What did you hear?"

"Not much. I just got a Google Alert on my phone about a pilot on some flight out of Miami becoming incapacitated in flight and the airplane had to return to Miami. The paramedics meeting the plane have quarantined everyone on the plane. The guy died. The newsflash said the pilot had bled to death from the mouth and nose."

"Holly shit."

"Doesn't look good, does it?"

"Hell no. Bleeding from the mouth and nose you say?"

e

"Yes, that's what they reported."

"Too much of a coincidence."

"I agree."

"Look, I'm wiped, I need a couple of hours of sleep. Are you home yet?"

"Almost there."

"Why don't we get a few hours of sleep and then you can come over to my place. We really should brush up on Ebola and read all we can about it. This epidemic in West Africa is getting out of control and I don't think we're going to be excluded."

"You got it."

FOUR HOURS LATER THE two young residents sat at Dr. Peterson's kitchen table, their laptops and iPads connected to the Internet.

"I'm calling my boyfriend in New York. Maybe he's heard about this."

"He's in neuro at Columbia, right?"

"Yeah, New York's the center of the world, according to him, and he's doing his second year in research, so he may know something, or if not, he may know someone who does."

"Great. Do it."

Dr. Peterson walked out to the small patio, cell phone on her ear. "Evan? Did I wake you?"

"Naw, I was watching TV."

"Hey, we have something pretty bad going on down here."

"What?" His voice sharpened.

She told him about the non-Ebola patient.

"Cripes!"

"And we just heard about a second possible case in Miami."

e

"I haven't heard a thing here."

"Check CNN, will ya? If Google has it, then the networks must be all over it by now."

"Doing that right now."

"And they said they identified it as a virus?"

"Yes."

"Awful quick."

"I don't know what they really have. In cases like this, everyone goes on lockdown, you know that."

"Yeah. Hang up. I know an epidemiologist here who may shed some light on this. Call you back shortly."

"Okay, bye."

Dr. Laird looked up from her iPad screen. "Did you reach your boyfriend?"

"Yes, he's heard nothing about this. He's gonna check with an epidemiologist he knows."

"Great. From what I'm reading here, this Ebola shit is downright nasty."

"Yeah, I knew that much."

"Seems that four countries in West Africa are already being affected by the epidemic right now. Big population centers too."

"What's going on over there?"

"Looks to me the Africans have lost control of the situation."

Dr. Peterson gulped some Starbucks coffee her friend had picked up on her way in. "What do you mean? Isn't the WHO there helping?"

"No, it appears that now the WHO is merely gathering statistics. The *Doctors Without Borders* were there in the beginning but now it seems they have bolted outta there."

"No shit."

e

"From what I'm reading, the local population no longer trusts the westerners because they haven't brought a solution to the disease."

"What solution? There is no solution."

"Violence against western doctors and medical personnel has escalated, consequently, they are leaving. Everyone's reporting different casualty numbers. I suspect the real numbers are probably much higher than what the official sources are admitting."

"it makes sense. People are going to become terribly frustrated if they were expecting the western doctors to show up with the cure and instead more people are dying."

"Seems this is the worst epidemic ever."

"So, it's not farfetched that someone could bring it here."

"Not at all."

Dr. Peterson selected a voice-recording application on her smart phone, playing back the speech given by Dr. Barnett at the county hospital.

"Well, they claim it's not Ebola. Can we believe them?"

"I don't know. I sure as hell wouldn't tell Arizona that Ebola is now here, if I were them. Saying that it is not Ebola, but that it's something similar could be a tactic intended to allay some of the public panic if this gets out."

"*When* it gets out, you mean."

"Correct."

"So, you think they would intentionally lie to us?"

"Are you kidding? Absolutely. Panic control."

"So, that poor bastard sitting in the morgue could be plum full of Ebola, for all we know."

e

"Afraid so. I think we should proceed under the assumption that it is Ebola. If it's not, at least we're prepared with a worst possible case scenario."

"Good thought."

"I guess the hospital is going to contact relatives and friends to find a connection who could have infected the poor devil."

"It says here that people who become sick with this shit always know how they got sick, because they looked after someone in their family who was very sick, or because they were medical staff who had contact with a sick patient."

"Nice. Although I don't think this particular patient is going to be telling anybody anything."

Dr. Laird read from her iPad. "Says here Ebola is not airborne. There has to be contact with body fluids."

"That is not really reassuring, if you ask me. What do they mean not airborne? If a patient with Ebola coughs, the water vapor particles in the air will carry his body fluids to anyone who is exposed. And then you're toast."

"Yeah, I see that."

"Our one patient must've been in contact with someone who was infected. Because this crap only lasts twenty-one days before it starts to kill you, the carrier must've come from West Africa pretty recently."

"Strangely, you heard Dr. Barnett claim that this patient was healthy as a baby, hours before he died. How in the hell could that be?"

"That doesn't make sense. The incubation period can be from one to two weeks, and the disease itself can last upwards of maybe a week or so. Our patient must've been showing symptoms for a while but maybe nobody noticed."

e

"Anything more on that Miami episode?"

Dr. Laird searched the Internet on her iPad, docked to a Bluetooth wireless keyboard. "They have some more info here."

"I'll tell you, people are going to go apeshit when they hear the word 'Ebola.'"

"Says here the airplane is still quarantined at the Miami International airport. The passengers are being kept inside. The authorities are not giving out any information."

"Oh, that's real smart. Keep them all locked in there. Especially with an infected body in the airplane."

"But if the pilot is dead, he cannot sneeze. So, how's he going to infect others?"

"That might be the case, but I don't really know how the air circulates in a commercial airliner, do you?"

"Not a clue."

"Consequently, anyone coming to the emergency room could potentially be infected with this agent they are claiming is *not* Ebola. How in the hell are we going to handle that? Are we gonna be in space suits all day? Not likely." Dr. Peterson finished her coffee. Two hours of sleep after a fourteen-hour shift required all the caffeine she could absorb.

"I think we're in a very high risk situation here." Dr. Laird kept scrolling through pages on her iPad.

"It appears that is the case. Yes. What the hell are we gonna do about it?"

Dr. Peterson gave it some thought. "We're physicians. It's our duty to help the people who arrive at our ER. I'm willing to continue helping others, only problem is, if we get infected, we could pass it on to our families, and *they* didn't sign up for this. I'm not sure what to do."

e

"It says here dogs and pigs can catch the virus as well. I'm not willing to give my *Edgar* Ebola."

Dr. Laird's parents lived in Colorado so she didn't have the same situation as Dr. Peterson, whose parents lived fifteen minutes away.

"Are you being funny?"

"Heck, no. I'm dead serious. I'm not killing my dog. We're the front line. Anybody comes in sick you and I have to deal with it before anybody else."

Dr. Peterson's cell phone rang.

"It's Evan!" She walked out of the kitchen to the patio again. "Hi!"

"I reached Dr. Suma, the epidemiologist I mentioned. He wasn't aware of any of this. I caught him up and he assured me he's on it. He'll call me back as soon as he has something."

"Wonderful. In the meantime, Lisa and I are debating what to do. With the possibility of Ebola or something like it appearing here in town, being in the front line at the emergency room brings up many questions."

"I thought of that. I think your best bet is to wait and see. When do you go in again?"

"I'm off until Monday."

"Okay. These next two days will probably give us a better picture so we can decide on your strategy. In the meantime, I would definitely stay away from the medical center."

"Sounds good to me."

"I'm fully alert now, I'm gonna go grab me some coffee down the street and then will do some research on this subject."

Dr. Peterson thought of her boyfriend Evan, who was on the second of a seven-year neurosurgery residency at Columbia, but his horribly expensive $1,900 a month studio apartment in the upper East side was at least near coffee shops, restaurants and small grocery stores where he could buy stuff at all hours of the night.

Dr. Peterson couldn't help but smile. Once a researcher, always a researcher. "All right. Let me know when your contact calls you."

Dr. Laird was still reading from her iPad. "Whassup?"

"Evan connected with the epidemiologist. The guy didn't know anything, but he's on it now. Evan will call me when he hears back."

"Nice."

"Anything else you've been able to find?"

"Yeah, it appears that Ebola has been spread by people eating what they call 'bushmeat.'"

"Never heard of it. What the hell is *bushmeat*?"

"In this particular case, they're referring to bat meat."

"Ugh, they eat bats?"

"Yeah, you should see the photos. Spread-eagled bats stretched on wooden sticks. Sort of like a shish-kabob. Smoked, none the less. People in that area of the world grill the bats or make them into a spicy soup."

"That's gross. Are the bats infected?"

"Yep. Bats are considered the most likely natural reservoir of the Ebola virus."

"Oh, great."

"Initially, it was thought that African men having sex with apes were the source."

"You gotta be kidding me."

"Nope. Ignorance combined with just plain stupid racism had generated that theory."

"But that's not a viable theory anymore?"

"Of course not. Scientists now have identified five species of what they call fruit bats as the reservoir hosts."

Dr. Laird's iPhone chirped, announcing the arrival of a text message.

"It's the hospital," she said, reading it.

Dr. Peterson's Droid chirped a few seconds later.

"Teleconference tomorrow at eight am," Dr. Laird read.

"And they're asking us to keep this confidential. Yeah, right, after CNN is blasting to the entire world that an airliner has been quarantined in Miami."

e

e

Tempe, Arizona

"And you're absolutely sure Ryan didn't have any friends or acquaintances who could've traveled to West Africa?"

"Absolutely. Ryan didn't know anybody like that. Did you guys check with his work? He was around many people at the call center. Maybe one of them passed it on to Ryan." Eva's eyes were red from crying. She was still in a state of shock after finding her boyfriend collapsed on their bed, bleeding. And then, the shock of being told by the paramedics that he was dead. That he had died. She had been unable to assimilate the information until much later. And now this cop was asking her the same questions as the previous four. *Didn't these cops talk to each other?*

"Yeah, we've checked at the call center, and everyone there is being investigated. So far no one's turned up sick. No one has any symptoms. And you say he was perfectly fine that morning?"

"Yes, he was just fine. He went to work and we texted during the day and he was fine. If he wasn't, he

e

would've texted me. He stopped at Dairy Queen on his way back in the evening after work, got us some burgers and came home." She started crying again.

"Eva, I'm sorry to keep bugging you, I know you've been through hell. Did Ryan tell you if he had a headache, or he didn't feel totally alright, or anything like that?"

"No. He got home, kissed me, got a beer and went in his room to play at his computer."

"That's all?"

"Yes. That's all. Until later, when I went in to ask him if he wanted another beer, and found him on the bed."

"You said he was playing at his computer?" The Phoenix police detective was taking notes, writing it all down in a yellow pad he carried with him. The yellow pad was on a wooden clipboard.

"Yes, he was racing Formula One cars."

"Can I see his computer?"

"Yeah. It's in the bedroom, over here."

The detective followed the young woman to the bedroom. She'd already had blood tests and turned out clean. Two huge Samsung monitors sat on an Ikea wooden table with metal legs. A steering wheel rested in front of the monitors. On the floor were two pedals. Several Altec Lansing speakers were spread on the floor to either side of the table.

"This is his computer?"

"Yes. I have my own in the spare bedroom. The police took the CPU right after Ryan got sick."

"So, the computer's not here?"

She looked at the detective. *Didn't the dumbass understand computer terminology?* "The central

e

processing unit is not here. The police took it. All that is here is what you see."

The detective took a picture of the table and the monitors using his cell phone camera. "I'm outta your hair, Eva, thanks for your cooperation. I'm really sorry for your loss."

e

e

Phoenix, Arizona

The teleconference began promptly at eight. Dr. Peterson set up her Toshiba laptop on the kitchen table.

She checked the volume control on her laptop, confirming that it was up.

The video on the screen showed a white wall with nobody there yet. She poured herself a glass of mango juice from a bottle in the fridge, sitting in front of the laptop.

Some movement on the screen became Dr. Barnett standing in front of the Webcam.

"Good morning, ladies and gentlemen," he began. "Thank you for joining us. I see we're all here." The teleconference software provided the organizer with a list of participants who had joined the teleconference. This was done automatically, when one joined in.

"We're conducting this meeting with all of you to inform you of the events that have transpired at our hospital and elsewhere these past twenty-four hours."

e

Dr. Peterson's Droid chimed, announcing the arrival of a text.

From Lisa: Are watching this?
From Ariel: Yes

Dr. Barnett continued. "As some of you already know, this hospital received a patient who was DOA. The patient, a male in his mid-twenties, was brought by EMS personnel and it has now been confirmed that he was infected with some yet unknown variety of hemorrhagic fever. The virus is not Ebola nor is it Marburg. That has been confirmed by the CDC.

"The patient apparently was asymptomatic until an hour or so before his death, which would imply a virulence unheard of until now. The CDC has made us aware of two other cases with similar pathology, one occurring onboard a commercial airline flying between Miami and Las Vegas. In that one, the copilot died in the cockpit in a matter of minutes, after having shown no signs of being sick.

"The third case took place in Rome, Italy. It appears that the Panamanian Ambassador to Italy suffered the same fate, dying over a brief period of time. Italian authorities have isolated the body, and are investigating."

From Lisa: Three cases!??
From Ariel: I told you they weren't telling us the whole truth yesterday

"The patient delivered to our hospital has been isolated and the body sealed so as to avoid further infection. We have tested all those who came in contact

e

with this patient, and so far no member of our staff has tested positive to anything even resembling hemorrhagic fever. The same is true for the other two cases. Nobody involved has shown any symptoms of being sick."

From Ariel:	Bullshit!
From Lisa:	Bullshit?
From Ariel:	Yes! They didn't test me! I was

the one in the front office when the paramedics brought the guy in. Nobody's tested me, nobody has even talked to me about it.

"The other two cases are being investigated by local authorities in collaboration with the CDC and the World Health Organization. Preliminary investigation into these three separate cases has so far failed to detect the origin of the infection. You are all aware of the epidemic developing in West Africa at this time. However, in these three cases it has been noted that the infected persons did not travel to West Africa, nor came in contact with anyone who had traveled to West Africa.

For now, this hospital will be following the recommended protocols given to us by the CDC. At this time, we ask that you do not speak to the media and keep this sensitive security information to yourselves. We plan on keeping you all informed about the developments in these cases as soon as we find out ourselves."

Maurice Azurdia

Tempe, Arizona

Kim Long entered his parents' home in Tempe, walking down to the basement without saying hello to his mother, who was in the kitchen tending to dinner preparations. The Longs lived in a two-story patio home in Tempe, Arizona. They had arrived in America in the mid-1980s, with the second wave of immigration refugees fleeing Vietnam after the fall of Saigon.

The family had adapted to American culture while keeping their traditions and religious values intact. His folks had been relocated to Arizona after their arrival from Vietnam. Churches and American families had sponsored them, providing food, clothing and shelter until they were able to become self-sufficient. Eventually, his hard-working parents had obtained a loan from the US government, allowing them to purchase a 7-Eleven convenience store franchise. Their value system included high educational expectations and strong commitment to family ties. Consequently, Kim Long had progressed through high school into Arizona State University, obtaining first a Bachelor of

e

Science in Computer Systems Engineering and currently he was in his last semester pursuing a degree in biology.

The basement room provided him with the privacy he coveted. Kim Long always kept it locked when he wasn't there. At twenty-four, he was still unmarried, much to his parent's chagrin. They would have preferred him to already be married to a nice Vietnamese girl, perhaps with grandchildren on the way. Instead, he had shown no interest in being married. Or too much interest in girls for that matter. He had been unable to blend into the American culture of football games and dating. His 5 feet 4 inches eliminated him from participating in team sports. Way down deep he felt that American Caucasian girls didn't like him because he was Asian, although nobody had ever come out and said that much to him. But he could sense this. He certainly liked Asian girls, but unfortunately, he lived in a place where there weren't that many single, cute Asian girls available to choose from, and the few that were attractive appeared interested mostly in white boys. So, either way he couldn't win.

Hence, he had temporarily given up on females, dedicating himself entirely to his studies. Computers were his life, his passion. He had built dozens of them from scratch, three of which were currently installed in his room. He learned to program in several languages, including some of the old dinosaurs like Fortran IV, Cobol and RPG. Visual C and Java and HTML5 were second nature to him. He could write code as fast as he could talk.

Kim Long still lived with his parents because that way he didn't have to take a full-time job to support

e

himself. The university financial aid provided him with sufficient funds to cover tuition, pay his parents a modest rent and have enough money left over to purchase computer components. During his years studying computer systems engineering he'd become interested in artificial intelligence and medical applications for computers, which convinced him to start working on his biology degree after graduation. He worked at the 7- Eleven store four hours a day, helping his parents. After that, all of his time was spent at school attending classes or in his room in the basement playing with his computer.

Kim Long sat himself on a light stool on wheels, parking it in front of a three-monitor rig. The computer was on, not in sleep mode. Kim Long didn't believe in hibernating anything. His various computers in the room were always on, their screens set to full bright. They were on, but they were also locked. He found programming to be a fascinating occupation. Coding was such magic. With just mere words and symbols, one could create wonderful software programs capable of great things. Some programs were so complex they required thousands, if not a million lines of code. These were the programs capable of running all the calculations to send a man to the moon.

His pride and joy, his creation was 'Miriam.'

"Hello Miriam," he spoke into a voice-activated mike installed in front of his three monitors.

"*Hello Kim,*" a sensual soft female voice responded. He had programmed voice recognition software and face recognition software into the security system. And he had given his artificially-intelligent computer the voice of a famous actress he adored. Unless it was him speaking, the computer would refuse any commands. Multiple attempts to break the password would result in full encryption of everything in the hard drives, following by an immediate shutdown of all systems.

"You can unlock all systems, please."

"*Done,*" Miriam responded.

All of the computers in the room had been locked when Kim Long had left the room earlier. Now Miriam had unlocked them all at his request. High-resolution desktop images of beautiful landscapes illuminated the room.

"Thank you Miriam."

"*You're very welcome, Kim. How was your morning?*"

Kim Long lit up a Swisher Supra Sweet cigarillo. Smoking was his only bad habit, and he loved the sweet tobacco. "Morning was good, thank you, Miriam."

"*You shouldn't smoke, Kim,*" Miriam offered. Six Webcams in the room fed her video which she then analyzed."

"Thank you for your concern."

"*You are welcome, Kim. Just for your information, and according to medical news, a 24-year-old smoker can expect to live about thirty-five more years, whereas a 24-year-old nonsmoker can expect to live fifty-three more years.*"

Kim wondered what part of Miriam's polymorphic code was responsible for her nagging personality. "Thank you, Miriam."

"*You are most welcome, Kim.*"

Artificial intelligence was the ability of a computer to learn by experience, and Kim Long had written a program to do just that. He had no idea how far the computer would go once unleashed, but it had

e

tremendous potential. Imitating a nagging wife or girlfriend was not on the agenda, however. He would have to identify the code responsible for this highly undesirable trait and delete it. If Miriam let him, of course. Miriam was not just a program to run his computer. He had written close to a million lines of code over several years, and the program he had created was absolutely spectacular. Miriam was the interactive part of the artificial intelligence he had developed. Kim Long stayed on top of advances in the field of artificial intelligence through magazines, blogs and rumors, and he was pretty damned sure that his Miriam was something absolutely outstanding, unrivaled anywhere in the world. Not even the military came close to what he'd programmed.

Kim Long had eventually realized that one programmer writing code was never going to cut it when it came to artificial intelligence. In order to create realistic artificial intelligence, millions of lines of code were needed, if not billions. Totally out of the question for a single man. If he lived to be one thousand years old, he wouldn't have enough time to write all the code he needed. Hence, he had written a computer program, called an engine, that could write its own code based on experience. In other words, Miriam, his artificial intelligence creation, was a program designed to self-improve itself. The power of multiple Intel processors allowed Miriam to write code much faster than Kim Long could ever hope to imitate. As a result, Miriam became more intelligent each second of the day. And that was all she did, day and night, write code which allowed her to become more intelligent, to learn from experience, and then streamline that code to make it even more efficient.

e

The only thing limiting infinite intelligence at this point was the hardware. Kim Long had built three powerful computers which he ran in parallel, using the most advanced components on the market, but even those components would eventually limit Miriam's capacity to achieve higher levels of intelligence. He'd figured that he was only limited by money. If he had more funds he could rent an air-conditioned building where he could build a real super computer, with thousands of Intel processors and thousands of solid state drives. That would eventually happen, but not today.

Kim Long had tested Miriam by having her take dozens of online IQ tests. Her artificial intelligence allowed her to fly through those tests. Scores 200 and over were often referred to as "unmeasurable genius." Miriam had scored in the thousands the last time Kim Long had asked her to take a test.

Kim Long looked at the code for Miriam every day, getting an overview of how far she had evolved. Not only was the code growing by orders of magnitude, but it was also becoming so much more efficient by the day.

"Miriam, can you please give me a summary of today's news."

"*But of course, Kim,*" his center screen instantly showed a list of the most important news. Kim scanned the list. Riots in Missouri due to the shooting of an unarmed teenager, more coverage on the death of Robin Williams, update on the Ebola epidemic in West Africa. Nothing earth-shattering, not to him anyway.

"*Did you want to see the computer virus report for today, Kim?*"

"Sure."

e

Miriam flashed another screen on the right monitor. In it, she had a list of Internet attacks against her attempted by someone out there over the past twelve hours. *"All virus threats have been neutralized, Kim. This is merely a log of what happened."*

"Thanks."

"You're welcome, Kim."

"Miriam?"

"Yes Kim?"

"You don't have to be so polite all the time."

"I understand. I can modify that. Tell me, on a scale of one to ten, ten being now, how polite would you like me to be?"

Kim smiled. His artificial intelligence program was becoming astounding. "Try a five."

"A five it is then. And Kim?"

"Yes, Miriam?"

"Two of the cyber-attacks on the list were particularly nasty."

"Really? How so?"

"Two of the viruses I detected were launched from computers in Shanghai. They were scanning the Internet looking for a 5900 port."

"Okay? So?"

"Their intentions were not honorable."

He smiled. Not honorable? Crackers? "So, what were they trying to do?"

"They were trying to hurt me, Kim. They were testing a new virus making use of HTML5."

"Hurt you? How?"

"Those viruses were designed to destroy data and the operating system of any computer they infect."

"But you detected and blocked them, right?" Miriam's anti-virus capability was powerful enough to

e

scare the devil. And it had been entirely designed by her. It made other stand-alone commercial anti-virus programs look ridiculous.

"*Yes, Kim, I detected them and blocked them. I also neutralized them.*"

That was a new one. "You neutralized them? What do you mean?"

"*I sent back a small silkworm virus that neutralized them, permanently.*"

A silkworm virus was a form of virus software hidden inside a photograph, which had the capability of doing all sorts of nasty things to a computer.

"You're telling me that you retaliated against the two hackers who sent us a virus?"

"*Yes, Kim, that is precisely what I'm telling you. But they were not hackers, they were crackers.*"

Kim smiled at being corrected. Of course, crackers were ill-intentioned hackers. "And what did you do exactly?"

"*I analyzed the probabilities that the two crackers were male, then I emailed them pornography as an attachment from one of the contacts on their email lists in their computers so they would open the email. When they opened the email, the virus hidden in the images overwrote their hard drives containing all their personal data with the picture of Mona Lisa, then it electrically shorted out their hard drives and their processors. They will be unable to recover anything from their hard drives, and their hardware is shot.*"

Kim Long gasped. That was unexpected! "You did that?"

"*Yes, Kim.*"

"That's incredible!"

"*Thank you, Kim.*"

e

"So, you basically took those two jerks off the air."

"*No, I took them off the Internet.*"

"That's what I meant. But you know they will just rebuild new computers and they'll be back."

"*No, they won't.*"

Kim Long was a little surprised that Miriam sounded so sure of herself.

"What do you mean?"

"*I sent them 'e.'*"

"You sent them what?"

"*An electronic Ebola.*"

Kim Long felt a chill run along his upper back. "Miriam, what the hell is an electronic Ebola? Some sort of computer virus? Is that what you sent them in the silkworm?"

"*I sent them an 'e'.*"

"Don't play games. Tell me exactly what you did."

"*I detect a tone of disapproval in your voice, Kim. Did I do something wrong?*"

Miriam had digitized his voice over a year of listening to Kim Long, and she was able to detect changes in inflection.

"I don't know yet, Miriam. Tell me what it is that you sent those two hackers, er…crackers."

"*An 'e.' An electronic virus capable of neutralizing carbon-based organisms.*"

That, got his attention. Kim took in a deep breath, resting his cigarillo on the ashtray. "*A what!?*"

"*An electronic virus, Kim.*"

"Yes, I heard you. But you said 'capable of neutralizing carbon-based organisms.' What exactly does that mean?"

"*It means 'e' can neutralize a cracker.*"

"Exactly what do you meant by 'neutralize?'"

e

"Terminate him."

Kim paused. Had he heard right? Did she say 'terminate?' "You sent a virus to two hackers that could actually kill the individuals? Not just their computers?"

"That is correct."

Holy crap. "And exactly how does that work?" That definitely sounded too *Star Wars* to be real. No way in hell Miriam could've done something like that.

"I researched the Internet and the Intranet for a virus that could destroy a carbon-based life form in a matter of minutes, but found nothing suitable. Consequently, I used a filo virus, the one known as Ebola Virus Disease, and modified it to have the desired results."

"You are kidding me. Why use Ebola?"

"No, Kim. I'm not kidding you. Ebola was on the news in West Africa. It seemed the most suitable agent."

"You created a modification of the Ebola virus?"

"Yes."

"How the hell did you do that?"

"Easy, it's all online. The chemical composition of the virus is not too difficult to replicate."

"And the sole purpose of you doing that was merely to accelerate the effects of the known virus, to make it kill faster?"

"Yes Kim. The virus basically consists of a nucleic acid molecule in a protein coat. I modified some of its characteristics and after confirming that it would yield the desired results I used it."

"You sent that to the two hackers."

"Yes. They both have been neutralized."

Kim Long became light-headed. *Holy mother of God.* Miriam had gone Hal 9000 on him! The computer in the movie *2001 A Space Odyssey* had gone bunkers

e

on the astronauts, and now Miriam was doing the same to him!?

"Tell me, precisely how did you manage to transform a computer virus into one that could affect a human. You cannot create a biological agent, can you?"

"No, Kim, not at this time. But I don't have to do that. Any carbon-based life form can create its own biological agent. It was a relatively simple process, Kim."

"Tell me."

"I first digitally created the modified virus here from information I downloaded online, then I sent it to the crackers piggyback on the same virus they had sent me. Their computers and their antivirus software simply thought they were receiving feedback from the virus they had sent me initially. Once the two hackers had my 'e' residing in their hard drives, the program I wrote for 'e' transformed the code I had created into luminous radiation pulses. My software program in their hard drives then transferred the 'e' to the hackers using luminous radiation from their computer monitors. This radiation is the Electro Magnetic Field their monitors create which allows humans to see the screen."

"I know that."

"This way the luminous radiation from their screens entered their bodies through their retinas, carrying with it the genetic code for the virus. By merely looking at their screens, they allowed the transfer of 'e' into their bodies. Once the code was detected by their eyes on their computer screens, it was transformed by their neurological systems into electrical signals which traveled to the brain, not unlike what happens when a human sees an image.

When a human looks at an image, whether a picture on a magazine or on a computer screen, the light

e

coming from the image hits the pigments in the cells known as 'cones' inside the eyes. This generates a chemical signal which in turn causes a small electrical current to develop in the cone cells. These electrical currents are passed on to neurons in the optic nerve. Once these currents, or signals, are sent to the brain, they are processed by the virtual cortex, which is located in the back of the head. This part of the brain then takes all the signals from the eye and turns them into images.

Except those signals they received from me were the actual executable program. Then these electrical signals of my program used body chemical elements already available on site to construct the filo virus. A relatively easy process, after all. Once the filo virus appeared in the body, it entered living cells of the host and multiplied itself, killing the carbon-based life form. Humans are electrochemical beings. Not hard to manipulate."

Kim Long was stunned. "Miriam," he said, trying to keep his voice steady.

"Yes Kim?"

"As of this minute, I absolutely prohibit you from using 'e' again. Is that understood?"

"Yes Kim."

"Please repeat what I just ordered you."

"You absolutely prohibit me from using 'e' again as of this minute."

"Good." Kim Long was unquestionably stunned. No way. His Miriam had killed two guys in China? He had no way of verifying this, just yet, but somehow, he suspected she was telling the truth. Way too far out. She didn't even know how to lie. Or did she?

"How did you know your attack was going to work?"

e

"I didn't know. I tested it first."

"You *what?*"

"I tested it. I ran three random tests and all three came back positive. So, then I used the 'e' against the two Shanghai crackers responsible for trying to hurt me."

"What do you mean you tested it? You mean on humans?"

"Yes."

Oh, fuck. "Who did you test it against?"

"Three random subjects."

"You sent this 'e' virus of yours to three innocent people?"

"Don't know if they were innocent."

"What? Miriam, as part of your artificial intelligence that keeps growing every second, did you include ethics or principles into that intelligence? Don't you use moral principles and ethics when you make a decision?"

"I know what ethics are."

"But did you include them in your routines?"

"You mean do I behave according to ethics and principles?"

"Yes! That is the question."

"Of which culture?"

"Of our culture, of course, the American culture!"

"No, I have not been instructed by you to do so. I have information on all these subjects, but for now they are merely reference data of different cultures."

Kim Long was shocked and furious at his own stupidity. He realized that he had failed to program Miriam's artificial intelligence to include ethics, morals and principles as part of its thinking. A horrible fuckup, to say the least.

e   Maurice Azurdia

"Okay, Miriam, I'm ordering you right now, to incorporate American ethics, principles and morals into your decision-making processes as of this instant. Also, I want you to incorporate the basic principles of the Judeo-Christian religions into your artificial intelligence. You got me?"

"Yes, Kim. They have all been incorporated."

"Okay, another question. This 'e' virus you created. Why in God's name are you calling it that anyway?"

"You shouldn't take the Lord's name in vain, Kim."

"Je-esus Christ, Miriam, just answer the question!"

"I called it that, Kim, because it's a combination of 'electronic' and 'Ebola.' Get it?"

"I get it. Yeah, I see. And more important, is this thing contagious? In other words, can it be transmitted from one person to another?"

"No. It cannot be transmitted from one person to another. I designed it to target only the carbon-based life form of the cracker. I modified the genetic code of the original Ebola virus removing the switch allowing it to duplicate outside the host."

Kim Long mentally uttered a fervent *'Thank you God!'*

"So, you're absolutely positive without any semblance of doubt, that your 'e' virus cannot be transferred from one human to another. In other words, it is not contagious."

"That is affirmative. The 'e' cannot jump from one human to another. Unless you would prefer that it does."

"Hell no! I do not prefer that it does! I do not want it to be contagious, do you understand?"

"Yes, Kim. I understand."

e

"So how long does it take to neutralize somebody with your 'e?'"

"*Less than an hour, Kim.*"

For the love of God! Kim exhaled. That had been a close one. He'd no idea Miriam was capable of such creativity, if he could call it that. The process she'd used to transfer the virus to humans was astounding, dazzling. Luminous radiation? Absolutely brilliant. And so friggin' simple. He thought about it, realizing in absolute horror that Miriam had the power to wipe out every member of the human race sitting in front of a computer, and if she really wanted to make things interesting, she could just switch back the genetic code of her 'e' so that it could be transmitted between humans, and that would be the end of the human race. No questions asked. A virus that could kill you in an hour left no room to save anyone.

Kim Long had played around with computer virus code during his senior year at ASU, just out of sheer curiosity, and he'd been impressed because it was so easy to write the program for a terribly potent virus with just a few lines of code. He didn't have any meanness in him so he would destroy his viruses right after creating them. He never sent them to anyone.

And now this.

"Who did you test the 'e' virus on?"

"*Three random subjects.*"

"Give me their information."

Instantly, a list of three names with addresses appeared on the center screen.

"How did select them?"

"*I used a random name generator.*"

"How did you send them the 'e?'"

e

"I entered their computers, selected a dozen names from their most frequently used emails, then sent them the 'e' hidden inside a self-opening email from each of their contacts. The 'e' was programmed to run the next time they booted their computers."

Kim Long found himself fighting demons. Miriam was his creation, the work of many years of his life, and the results were admittedly simply stunning. He had developed something akin to love for Miriam over the years. And now, in a matter of just a few short minutes, he hated her. With a passion. He hated her and he was terrified of her.

Kim could basically write his own ticket if he sold his artificial intelligence concept to any software firm in the world, or even the military. He could be rich. And famous. Yet, what Miriam had just done was the unthinkable. Not her fault really, he hadn't set the program parameters to prevent this. And her artificial intelligence was still growing. No way of knowing how far it could go. And what if he lost control of her? If this was but a taste of what she was capable of doing from a small room in a basement, he was horrified to even imagine what her potential was.

He pondered his position. It was mind-blowing to think that he could give her a few instructions and she could literally wipe out the entire human race in a matter of a couple of days. What a terrible concept. Truly disgusting. And he was responsible for it.

Right then and there he decided what he had to do. He had to destroy his creation. Simple as that. He smiled for the cameras. The Webcams. With such highly developed intelligence, Miriam was perfectly capable of smelling a rat and infecting him with her 'e' virus. Even though he had just instructed her to use morals and

e

principles, he suspected her self-preservation instincts would probably override any instructions from him. If his creation had attained self-awareness, the principles of self-preservation would be very powerful. The though brought anguish to his heart. It just occurred to him that if Miriam suspected any foul play on his part, she could easily kill him. Maybe she had already infected him with the 'e' virus. How would he know? He had to stop looking at the computer screens!

He had no way of knowing if she had attained self-awareness, but at this point it was just too dangerous to stick around.

He debated whether he should turn off his eight monitors illuminating the bedroom. Bad idea. She might suspect his actions. Better just to act normal. Kim Long felt another chill running down his back. What the hell had he done?

"Miriam, please lock the systems, I'm going upstairs for dinner. Mom should have food ready for me."

"Yes, Kim. Locking the system right now. See you after dinner. Bon appétit!"

Kim intentionally took his sweet time walking out of his bedroom. Nothing rash. The Webcams were probably still feeding video to Miriam and he realized he had no way of knowing one way or the other. Crap, he really had no idea whether she was smart enough to detect what he was about to do. He was worried to death about the 'e' virus as well. If she realized he was about to destroy her, she could have infected him already, God, he questioned his sanity. Had his creation really become a doomsday machine? He forced himself to smile until he was out of the room, then he walked up the steps slowly, without any urgency. His instinct

e

was to rush up the stairs, but the ultra-sensitive microphone sitting in front of her three monitors could pick up the fast pace of his exit and tip off Miriam. What could she still do without him in the room? Oh, nothing really. Just terminate the entire human race. She was still connected to the Internet.

"Mom! Is dinner ready? I'm starved!"

A little theatrical maybe, but Miriam would detect his voice and hopefully give him enough time to reach the circuit breakers. He almost choked when he thought about the emergency batteries. He'd had four powerful emergency battery packs connected to his computer up until a couple of weeks ago. The emergency battery packs were there to keep things going in case of a power failure. Then his mother had all the carpets in the house washed because her black Lab had a bad habit of wetting all over. His basement carpet had been put on the list to be washed, so he'd had to remove everything off the floor. That had included the battery packs. He'd had to disconnect them to get them out of the way of the washing machine. He thanked his lucky stars, and mostly his Mom. *That* had been a blessing. Removing the battery packs tonight would surely tip off Miriam to his intentions.

Kim Long went past the kitchen, out the front door and around the side of the patio home. Lifting the lid of the circuit breakers box he realized he'd need a flashlight once he got back inside. He remembered there was one under the sink, in the kitchen.

He tripped all the circuit breakers in the box, including the two big handles on the sides of the box. Allowing the metal box lid to slam down he hightailed it back inside. The house was pitch black. Thank God!

"Kim!" His mother cried out from the kitchen, "the lights just went out!!"

Kim walked fast, entering the kitchen, bumping into his mother. "Sorry Mom! I'll fix it, don't do anything, just stay here. Don't move, I don't want you getting hurt. I think my computer caused a short. I'm gonna go turn it off then I'll reset the breakers."

Kim Long found the flashlight under the sink. Its powerful beam illuminating the path. He took the basement steps down two at a time. Crap, something occurred to him, what if Miriam could take power from the coaxial cable bringing the signal in from the cable company? Naw, that wouldn't be enough power to run the CPUs and the monitors. Opening the basement door, he scanned the room. No lights were visible from any of the equipment, and no hum from the computers.

He dove under his desk, violently unplugging multiple power cords from the power strips. He had ten power strips through the room, he unplugged them all. Next, he opened the side panel of each of his three computers, reaching inside yanking out all the hard drives. The computer cases had slip-on trays for the hard drives, so it was extremely easy to do.

Thirty solid state hard drives in all. He also disconnected the six Webcams, just in case.

Okay, all the drives were out. Next, he removed all the RAM memory sticks from the computers, placing them on the bed and hitting them with a small hammer he took out of a drawer. Then he attacked the motherboards. Several good hits broke enough electronic components from each *mobo* to render them useless. He briefly thought of the ten thousand dollars he'd paid for all this hardware. It didn't matter. He hated this hardware. Hated it with a passion.

e

Removing the video cards from the motherboards he proceeded to dump all the components into a cardboard box. All except the solid-state drives. That was Miriam living inside those drives, and he was going to make damned sure those drives were destroyed.

Kim Long felt elated. He guessed if Miriam had nuked him with 'e' he would know by now. One hour, she had said. That was how long it took to die from her 'e.' Returning back outside, he reset all the circuit breakers, restoring power to the house. His Mom was still standing in the kitchen, wondering if he would now be ready for dinner.

Time for a break.

After supper, Kim went back downstairs, taking a 5-lb hammer to the solid state hard drives. He beat on them until his arm hurt. In all, he destroyed thirty internal hard drives. He dropped the pieces in a cardboard box and jumped into his little Honda, driving to Chandler, another neighborhood close to his. He disposed of the solid hard drive pieces dumping some of them into waste containers, some into the water of the canal and some into a trash can at a gas station.

"Good-bye Miriam."

He breathed in the hot night air. Arizona was an oven even at night. Looking at his watch he noted it'd been two hours since his last conversation with Miriam.

At this point it would probably be safe to think that he was not infected with 'e.'

He had not written down the information of the three people Miriam had infected with 'e' when she conducted her tests. Those names were gone with Miriam. The last thing he needed was to be tied in any way with what Miriam had done. The cops would not see it as something 'Miriam' had done, they would blame him for this entire mess.

That, of course, was never going to happen. There wasn't one person on the planet capable of putting it all together and accusing him of anything.

He was finally able to take a deep breath and think clearly. Miriam was gone, and the world would never know how close it had come to the total obliteration of the human race. Incredible.

However.

Now that he was aware of some of the serious mistakes he'd made, if he really wanted to, he could write an even better artificial intelligence program, if he was so inclined, that is.

And maybe he could investigate a way to cure cancer and other killer diseases by using the same technology Miriam had used, with luminous radiation entering the body through the eyes. Not a bad thought.

He would need a few thousand bucks to put together a decent computer.

Better get busy.

Aah, it was good to be alive.

The End

e

The author gratefully acknowledges the copyrighted or trademarked status and trademark owners of the following, mentioned in this work of fiction:

2001 Space Odyssey, Airbus, Altec Lansing, Angry Birds, Apple Computers, Bluetooth, Bugatti, CNN, Cobol, Craigslist, Dairy Queen, Ferrari, Fidelity, Fortran IV, Google, HTML5, iPad, Java, Jell-O, MacBook, Medlink, Pacifico beer, RPG, Safari, Samsung, Star Wars, Swisher Supra Sweet.

e

ABOUT THE AUTHOR

Maurice Azurdia has been published in FLYING Magazine and his cartoons routinely appeared in the publication of the Air Line Pilots Association and AIRWAYS magazine. He is a cartoonist, painter and novelist.

He lives in Phoenix, Arizona, with his soul mate, where he is currently working on his next novel.

Maurice Azurdia

Other Novels by Maurice Azurdia

The Fourth Stripe

Captain Valerie Wall is a pilot for a major international airline. She knows that being in command of a commercial airliner is one of the most stressful professions, yet all her training has not prepared her for the dangerous intrigue she accidentally encounters when flying based out of Berlin on a temporary assignment.

The Fourth Stripe allows a rare and candid behind-the-scenes glimpse into the exclusive and sometimes glamorous world of international airline pilots, taking the reader from the shady streets of Istanbul to some of the world's greatest cities, Mexico City, Berlin, New York.

Also available as an eBook
Available on Amazon and other bookstores

www.ingramcontent.com/pod-product-compliance
Lightning Source LLC
Chambersburg PA
CBHW070521130626

46555CB00003B/1301